UVEITIS NUTRITION FOR NEWLY DIAGNOSED

Optimize Your Diet To Combat Inflammation, Support Immunity, Alleviate Symptoms, Protect Vision, And Enhance Wellness

DR. ERIC TRISTAN

CONTENTS

Copyright © 2024, By Dr. Eric Tristan

DISCLAIMER

The information provided in this book, is intended for informational purposes only. The content is not intended to be a substitute for professional medical advice, diagnosis, or treatment. Always seek the advice of your physician or other qualified health provider with any questions you may have regarding a medical condition. Never disregard professional medical advice or delay in seeking it because of something you have read in this book.

The author of this book has made reasonable efforts to ensure that the information provided is accurate and up-to-date at the time of publication. However, the author makes no representations or warranties of any kind, express or implied, about the completeness, accuracy, reliability, suitability, or availability of the information contained within these pages.

Any reliance you place on the information provided in this book is strictly at your own risk. The author shall not be liable for any loss, injury, or damage arising from the usc of this book or the information contained herein.

The mention or reference to any individuals, products, websites, organizations, or other names within this book does not imply endorsement by the author. The inclusion of such references is solely for informational purposes and does not constitute an endorsement or recommendation.

Furthermore, the author disclaims any association or affiliation with any individuals, products, websites, organizations, or other names mentioned in this book.

It is important to consult with a qualified healthcare professional before making any dietary or lifestyle changes, especially if you have a medical condition. Each individual's health situation is unique, and what works for one person may not work for another.

Again, the information provided in this book is not intended to diagnose, treat, cure, or prevent any disease or health condition. Always seek the advice of a physician or other qualified health provider regarding any medical questions or concerns you may have.

Thank you for your understanding and for taking the necessary precautions when considering the information presented in this book.

ABOUT THIS BOOK

An indispensable and all-encompassing resource, "Uveitis Nutrition" examines the crucial convergence of nutrition and the management of uveitis. This book commences with a scholarly Introduction that establishes the foundation for a more comprehensive examination of the intricacies of uveitis and the possible consequences of dietary decisions. The Overview of Uveitis establishes a fundamental comprehension for readers by explicating the importance of being informed about this inflammatory condition of the eye.

An exploration of the critical role that nutrition plays in the management of previous is the subject matter of this book. The following chapters delve into the nutritional constituents and their influence on uveitis, with a particular focus on the correlation between dietary decisions and inflammation. The Anti-inflammatory Diet for Uveitis provides readers with a pragmatic manual that elucidates dietary adjustments that can effectively mitigate symptoms.

This book provides a comprehensive analysis of the importance of Key Vitamins and Minerals, emphasizing their function in promoting eye health. The influence of omega-3 fatty acids, which are acknowledged for their anti-inflammatory characteristics, is investigated concerning uveitis. An exclusive segment devoted to "Foods to Include and Foods to Avoid in the Uveitis Diet" offers practical recommendations for those in search of dietary direction.

Following a discussion of the significance of hydration in uveitis, the function of antioxidants in uveitis prevention is investigated. A comprehensive analysis is conducted on dietary supplements intended to support uveitis, providing a profound comprehension of supplementary approaches to managing the condition. The implications of lifestyle factors on uveitis highlight the comprehensive methodology espoused in this book.

Acknowledging the importance of individualized guidance, this book provides readers with a systematic approach to nutrition through consultation with a nutritionist or dietitian. Particulate Nutrition Plans for Patients Afflicted with Uveitis Offer feasibly implemented dietary modification strategies. Case Studies on Uveitis and Nutrition provide tangible illustrations from the real world, thereby strengthening the practical relevance of nutritional interventions.

In conclusion, this book delves into forthcoming trends in uveitis nutrition research, emphasizing its dedication to remaining updated on emergent developments. In summary, "Uveitis Nutrition" provides a comprehensive understanding of the critical role nutrition plays in managing this intricate ocular condition, making it an essential resource for nutritionists, healthcare professionals, and individuals impacted by uveitis.

CHAPTER ONE

Introduction

Uveitis, a severe ocular condition distinguished by inflammation of the uvea (consisting of the ciliary body, choroid, and iris), is capable of causing vision impairment or even total blindness if not effectively controlled. Due to the genetic and environmental components of uveitis, which contribute to its multifactorial nature, its treatment is frequently complex and requires a holistic approach. Nutrition is an area that is receiving growing attention in the management of uveitis. The significance of nutrition in facilitating holistic well-being is widely acknowledged, and recent studies indicate that particular dietary selections may be instrumental in mitigating the symptoms of uveitis and advancing ocular health.

A Synopsis Of Uveitis

Before discussing the function of nutrition in the management of uveitis, it is critical to have a thorough understanding of the condition. Uveitis is a collective term denoting a cohort of inflammatory disorders that impact the uvea, rather than being a singular disease. This inflammation may manifest in various ocular regions, resulting in a variety of symptoms including pruritus, discomfort, sensitivity to light, and impaired visual acuity. Idiopathic uveitis or uveitis associated with systemic conditions such as infections or autoimmune disorders may occur.

The diagnosis and treatment of uveitis pose significant challenges due to its intricate nature. Traditional methods incorporate immunosuppressive medications and corticosteroids, both of which have the potential to induce adverse effects and exhibit limited efficacy.

Consequently, healthcare professionals and researchers are investigating supplementary approaches, such as nutrition, to enhance the efficacy of uveitis management.

Nutritional Importance In Uveitis Management

Supporting the immune system and maintaining overall health are both dependent on proper nutrition. When considering uveitis, it is possible that a nutrient-dense and nutritionally balanced diet could influence the inflammatory response, diminish oxidative stress, and facilitate the body's innate healing mechanisms. Uveitis and numerous chronic diseases share the characteristic of inflammation, and specific dietary constituents have been recognized for their potential anti-inflammatory attributes.

Furthermore, uveitis is frequently linked to autoimmune disorders, and empirical data indicates that dietary components may impact the response of the immune system. As a result, a customized nutritional strategy can enhance conventional therapies and contribute to a more all-encompassing approach to managing uveitis.

The Effects Of Dietary Components On Uveitis

1. Anti-inflammatory Nutrients: Since inflammation is a major cause of uveitis, its effects can be mitigated by consuming anti-inflammatory nutrients. Omega-3 fatty acids, which are present in walnuts, fatty fish, and flaxseeds, have exhibited anti-inflammatory characteristics. These lipids possess the ability to regulate the inflammatory response of the body and potentially aid in the mitigation of inflammation linked to uveitis.

2. Antioxidants are crucial in the prevention of uveitis and other ocular diseases associated with oxidative stress. By neutralizing free radicals, antioxidants—which are present in fruits, vegetables, and nuts—can mitigate oxidative stress. Minerals such as selenium and zinc, in addition to vitamins A, C, and E, are essential for preserving ocular health and bolstering the antioxidant defense system.

3. Anti-Angiogenic Foods: Angiogenesis, an abnormal proliferation of blood vessels caused by

inflammation, can be induced by uveitis. Anti-angiogenic properties are associated with green tea, dark chocolate, and foods abundant in resveratrol (which is present in fruits and red wine). By incorporating these into the diet, uveitis may be better managed and angiogenesis in the eyes may be better regulated.

4. Immune-Modulating Nutrients: Uveitis frequently involves dysregulation of the immune system. Fortified dairy products and oily fish both contain vitamin D, which is an essential nutrient for immune modulation. Potential benefits of maintaining sufficient vitamin D levels include immune response regulation and possible alleviation of the severity of uveitis symptoms.

5. The adoption of dietary patterns that prioritize whole foods, including lean proteins, fruits, vegetables, and whole cereals, offers a diverse array of nutrients that are advantageous for the overall well-being of an individual.

Those afflicted with uveitis may find the anti-inflammatory properties of a Mediterranean-style diet to be especially advantageous. Olive oil, fish, almonds, and an abundance of fruits and vegetables are all components of this diet.

In summary, although nutrition should not serve as a substitute for traditional medical interventions in the management of uveitis, it can offer a supplementary function. Incorporating a diverse and nutritious diet that is abundant in antioxidants and anti-inflammatory foods could potentially aid in the mitigation of inflammation, fortification of the immune system, and enhancement of ocular well-being.

Patients diagnosed with uveitis ought to seek guidance from healthcare practitioners, such as registered dietitians, to formulate individualized nutrition plans that are consistent with their comprehensive treatment approaches. The incorporation of nutrition into the paradigm of uveitis management has the potential to improve the visual outcomes and overall health of individuals afflicted with this difficult ocular condition.

A Uveitis Anti-Inflammatory Diet

A condition known as uveitis, which is distinguished by inflammation of the uvea (including the choroid, ciliary body, and iris), an anti-inflammatory diet may be beneficial. Embracing an anti-inflammatory dietary regimen potentially aids in symptom management and promotes optimal eye health as a whole.

The central tenet of an anti-inflammatory diet is the restriction of pro-inflammatory foods and the promotion of those that possess anti-inflammatory properties. This entails integrating an assortment of foods that are abundant in nutrients and are recognized for their capacity to mitigate inflammation. An omega-3 fatty acid, phytochemical, and antioxidant-rich diet is indispensable for preventing inflammation.

Essential Minerals And Vitamins For Uveitis

Specific vitamins and minerals are of paramount importance in promoting ocular well-being and regulating the inflammation that is linked to uveitis. Sufficient consumption of these nutrients may positively impact the overall health of the eyes.

Vitamin A is indispensable for the preservation of corneal health and the prevention of night blindness, an accompanying symptom of uveitis. Due to its antioxidant properties, vitamin C aids in the protection of the eyes against oxidative stress. Additionally, vitamin E may possess anti-inflammatory and immune-boosting properties.

Additionally, minerals such as selenium and zinc are vital for ocular health. Zinc is involved in the preservation of the structural integrity of eye tissues, whereas the anti-inflammatory properties of selenium contribute to this process.

CHAPTER TWO

Omega-3 Fatty Acids For Uveitis

The anti-inflammatory properties of omega-3 fatty acids, specifically eicosapentaenoic acid (EPA) and docosahexaenoic acid (DHA), may prove advantageous in the treatment and management of uveitis. The aforementioned foods contain these vital fatty acids: fatty fish, flaxseeds, chia seeds, and walnuts.

Omega-3 fatty acids may aid in the reduction of inflammation throughout the body, including in the eyes, according to scientific research.

By modulating the production of inflammatory molecules, they can enhance the equilibrium of the immune response. Omega-3 fatty acids are abundant in salmon, mackerel, and sardines, among other fish that can be incorporated into the diet.

Incorporating Foods Into A Uveitis Diet

A diet that is conducive to uveitis should give precedence to foods that possess anti-inflammatory and eye-supportive attributes. Aside from antioxidants, dark leafy greens such as kale and spinach are abundant in vitamins A, C, and E. Carrots, citrus fruits, and berries are examples of colorful fruits and vegetables that contribute to a balanced nutrient profile.

As previously stated, fatty fish are a remarkable reservoir of omega-3 fatty acids. Nuts and seeds, flaxseeds and walnuts in particular, are rich in omega-3 fatty acids and other vital nutrients. Fiber, which is present in legumes and whole grains, promotes general well-being and potentially exerts indirect anti-inflammatory influences.

Foods Excluded From The Uveitis Diet

While specific foods may provide benefits for uveitis, others have the potential to worsen inflammation and should be restricted or avoided.

The consumption of processed foods that are rich in trans fats and refined carbohydrates may promote inflammation and oxidative stress. Potential benefits include a reduction in the consumption of fried foods, sugary munchies, and processed proteins.

Additionally, excessive caffeine and alcohol consumption should be limited, as they may exacerbate inflammation. Some individuals with uveitis may experience increased inflammation due to dairy sensitivity; therefore, individuals with this condition may wish to restrict their dairy consumption.

In summary, it is imperative to embrace a nutritionally balanced regimen that prioritizes anti-inflammatory foods and vital nutrients to effectively manage uveitis. Adhering to a diet abundant in antioxidants, vitamins, and minerals has the potential to promote optimal eye health and mitigate inflammation-related symptoms. Although dietary modifications should not be regarded as a substitute for medical treatments advised by healthcare practitioners, they can serve as a valuable supplementary strategy in the management of uveitis and the advancement of sustained ocular health. It is strongly advised to seek guidance from a registered dietitian or a healthcare professional before implementing substantial dietary modifications, particularly if one has a pre-existing medical condition.

Moisturization And Uveitis

A group of inflammatory eye conditions that affect the uvea, the middle layer of the eye, is referred to as uveitis. Although pharmacological and medical interventions are frequently employed in the treatment of uveitis, adequate hydration should not be disregarded. Sufficient hydration is an essential component in preserving overall well-being and may have an indirect influence on ocular health, encompassing conditions such as uveitis.

Adequate hydration is crucial for immune system support, and a healthy immune system is indispensable for the management of inflammation, which is a defining characteristic of uveitis.

Water is a vital substance that facilitates the transportation of oxygen, nutrients, and immune cells across the entire body, thereby supporting the optimal operation of all organs, including the eyes.

The efficacy of the immune system may be compromised by dehydration, which has the potential to worsen the inflammatory responses that are linked to uveitis.

Additionally, maintaining adequate hydration is crucial for preserving the body's fluid balance and averting complications like dehydrated eyes. Uveitis patients frequently experience dry eyes; protecting against dehydration alleviates this discomfort.

Hydration management for uveitis entails consuming an adequate quantity of water daily. While individual recommendations may differ, a basic principle is to ensure adequate hydration by consuming a minimum of eight 8-ounce containers of water daily. This can be modified by variables such as climate, age, and level of physical activity.

In brief, hydration plays a critical role in the management of uveitis by promoting general well-being and enhancing the body's capacity to tolerate inflammation.

CHAPTER THREE

Antioxidant Function In Uveitis Prevention

Antioxidants are of the utmost importance in the prevention and management of numerous health conditions, such as uveitis. Anterior uveitis is characterized by inflammation of the eye, and the progression of inflammatory diseases is frequently associated with oxidative stress. Antioxidants mitigate oxidative stress through the neutralization of detrimental free radicals, consequently suppressing inflammation and promoting optimal eye well-being.

In addition to minerals such as zinc and selenium, vitamins C and E are potent antioxidants recognized for their ability to safeguard ocular tissues. Antioxidants contribute to the preservation of the eye's blood vessels, tissues, and cells. Moreover, they provide immune system support, thereby aiding in the regulation of inflammation within the body.

Vegetables and fruits are abundant in antioxidants. An assortment of vibrantly colored produce that is consumed offers a spectrum of antioxidants that may have preventative effects against uveitis. The antioxidant content of leafy greens, citrus fruits, berries, and seeds makes them suitable for incorporation into a balanced diet.

Omega-3 fatty acids, which are abundant in flaxseeds and oily fish such as salmon, also possess antioxidant and anti-inflammatory properties. Consuming these nutrients could potentially aid in the management of inflammation that is linked to uveitis.

Although incorporating antioxidants into one's diet can be advantageous, it is crucial to seek guidance from a healthcare professional to ascertain specific requirements and the possibility of requiring supplements. Supplements may be suggested in certain circumstances where dietary modifications alone fail to supply adequate levels of antioxidants, thereby augmenting the protective effects.

In summary, antioxidants play a crucial role in the prevention of uveitis by mitigating oxidative stress and inflammation, thereby promoting optimal eye health.

Supportive Dietary Supplements For Uveitis

Dietary supplements may lend a supportive capacity to the management of uveitis when utilized in conjunction with a balanced cuisine. It is imperative to seek guidance from a healthcare professional before integrating supplements into one's regimen. However, specific nutrients have exhibited the potential to promote ocular well-being and mitigate inflammation linked to uveitis.

Omega-3 fatty acids, which are frequently present in fish oil supplements, may be beneficial to uveitis patients due to their anti-inflammatory properties. Omega-3 supplementation may potentially mitigate the inflammatory response and prevent the recurrence of uveitis episodes, according to studies.

Eletromines, zinc, vitamin D, and selenium, among others, are vital for immune function and may aid in the treatment of uveitis. Deficiencies in vitamin D, which is specifically involved in the regulation of the immune system, have been associated with autoimmune disorders, including those that impact the eyes.

Foods containing the flavonoid quercetin, such as pears, berries, and scallions, contain antioxidant and anti-inflammatory properties. Some studies indicate that quercetin supplementation might be able to alleviate inflammatory responses in uveitis, although further research is required.

It is crucial to emphasize that supplements ought to be utilized in conjunction with a balanced diet, not instead of it. Utilizing supplements excessively or exclusively may result in unfavorable consequences. For the determination of the optimal dosage and combination of supplements that are customized to an individual's requirements, professional guidance is essential.

In summary, specific nutritional supplements may be incorporated into a holistic strategy for the management of uveitis, bolstering the immune and anti-inflammatory systems of the body.

Factors In Lifestyle And Uveitis

Numerous lifestyle factors, in addition to nutrition, can impact the progression and treatment of uveitis. Several lifestyle factors, including nicotine, stress, and sleep patterns, can affect ocular health.

Prolonged stress has the potential to impair the immune system and promote inflammation, both of which may serve as triggers or exacerbators for episodes of uveitis. Implementing stress management strategies, such as engaging in regular exercise, yoga, or meditation, can yield positive outcomes by bolstering the body's capacity to regulate inflammation and enhance general wellness.

Sufficient rest is a critical component of overall well-being, encompassing ocular health. Sleep is essential for the restoration and regeneration of the eyes; therefore, inadequate rest may contribute to inflammation and eye pain. Implementing regular sleep schedules may have a beneficial effect on the management of uveitis.

A well-established risk factor for numerous eye conditions, including uveitis, is smoking. Uveitis symptoms may be exacerbated by the oxidative stress and inflammation in the eyes caused by the toxic compounds in tobacco smoke. It is essential to refrain from smoking or minimize residual smoke exposure to preserve ocular health.

In addition, routine ocular examinations and timely identification of uveitis symptoms are critical for effective treatment and intervention.

Those who have a family history of uveitis or autoimmune conditions should exercise heightened caution and proactivity when it comes to monitoring their eye health.

In summary, lifestyle factors exert a substantial influence on the management of uveitis. By prioritizing sleep, addressing stress, and abstaining from smoking, individuals can enhance their overall eye health and potentially improve their ability to prevent or manage uveitis.

Managing Inflammation

A group of inflammatory eye diseases that affect the uvea, uveitis can have a substantial effect on vision and eye health as a whole. Although medical interventions such as immunosuppressive medications and steroids are crucial in the management of uveitis, the significance of nutrition in reducing inflammation and promoting general health should not be underestimated.

Therefore, individuals with uveitis must consult a nutritionist or dietitian to develop individualized nutrition plans that are specifically designed to address their unique requirements.

A Consultation With A Dietitian Or Nutritionist:

The collaboration between nutrition professionals and uveitis patients is increasingly acknowledged as a fundamental component of holistic healthcare. Nutritionists and dietitians are qualified to evaluate an individual's dietary patterns, way of life, and particular health issues to develop individualized recommendations for uveitis management that rectify nutritional deficiencies.

A nutritionist will customarily perform a comprehensive evaluation of the patient's dietary patterns throughout the consultation, identifying possible avenues for enhancement and assessing the intake of essential nutrients. Patients diagnosed with uveitis frequently encounter difficulties associated with inflammation and oxidative stress. In such cases, the assistance of a nutritionist can be beneficial in the selection of foods that are abundant in antioxidants and anti-inflammatory compounds. Fatty fish, flaxseeds, and walnuts contain omega-3 fatty acids, which have demonstrated anti-inflammatory properties and may provide potential benefits for individuals with uveitis.

Furthermore, nutritionists can inform patients regarding the inflammatory effects of specific foods. An illustration of this is a diet that is abundant in saturated fats and refined carbohydrates, which may promote inflammation and worsen the symptoms of uveitis. Dietary balance, consisting of a variety of lean proteins, fruits, vegetables, and whole carbohydrates, is the objective of nutritionists, who seek to establish an anti-inflammatory milieu within the body.

CHAPTER FOUR

Personalized Dietary Plans For Patients With Uveitis

The etiology of uveitis is multifactorial, and as a result, patients' nutritional requirements can vary considerably. Personalized nutrition regimens consider individual characteristics, including but not limited to age, gender, and pre-existing health conditions, in addition to the severity and type of uveitis.

In individualized nutrition regimens for patients with uveitis, addressing potential nutrient deficiencies is a crucial component. Certain nutrients, including zinc and selenium, as well as vitamins A, C, and E, are vital for maintaining healthy eyes and a robust immune system. Nutritionists possess the ability to suggest particular foods or supplements that guarantee a sufficient consumption of said nutrients.

Additionally, dietary triggers must be taken into account when attempting to manage uveitis symptoms. Specific food items may provoke allergic reactions or exacerbate inflammation, thereby exacerbating the condition. Using meticulous assessment and surveillance, nutritionists possess the ability to assist individuals in recognizing and eradicating potential dietary triggers, thereby enhancing the overall management of symptoms.

Pupils with uveitis should incorporate anti-inflammatory items into their individualized nutrition regimens as a fundamental component. An assortment of vibrant fruits and vegetables, turmeric, ginger, and green tea are recognized for their anti-inflammatory attributes. Patients can receive guidance from nutritionists on how to integrate these foods into their dietary regimens to enhance overall health and reduce inflammation.

Advancements In Uveitis Nutrition Research In The Future

With the continuous advancement of knowledge regarding the complex correlation between nutrition and uveitis, present and forthcoming scientific pursuits strive to elucidate more targeted dietary interventions that may serve as supplementary approaches to conventional treatments. Potential benefits of nutrigenomics, which investigates the impact of individual genetic variations on nutrient responses, include the ability to customize dietary regimens to the specific genetic composition of each individual.

Additionally, scientists investigate the function of the gastrointestinal microbiome in uveitis. The gut-brain-eye axis posits that ocular inflammation might be influenced by gastrointestinal health. The potential of probiotics, prebiotics, and dietary interventions that promote a healthy gut microbiome in the management of uveitis is currently under investigation.

Moreover, ongoing research is dedicated to the advancement of targeted nutritional supplements that are specifically formulated for patients with uveitis. These dietary supplements may contain bioactive compounds and nutrients that possess anti-inflammatory and antioxidant properties. Their purpose is to offer a practical and efficient supplement to traditional treatments.

In summary, uveitis nutrition necessitates a comprehensive strategy that incorporates personalized nutrition plans, collaboration with nutrition experts, and continuous investigation into the complex interrelationships between dietary patterns and ocular well-being. With the ongoing advancement of knowledge regarding uveitis and its nutritional ramifications, the incorporation of nutrition into the comprehensive management approach may have the capacity to improve the health and quality of life of those afflicted with the condition.

Conclusion

In summary, nutrition is an essential factor in the management of uveitis, an inflammatory condition that has the potential to impair vision and impact the eye.

There is scientific evidence indicating that specific nutrients have the potential to affect the immune response and inflammatory mechanisms, thereby influencing the severity and progression of uveitis. Minerals and antioxidants, including zinc and omega-3 fatty acids, as well as vitamins A, C, and E, have demonstrated potential in mitigating inflammation and promoting ocular well-being.

A nutritionally balanced diet that is abundant in fruits, vegetables, whole cereals, and lean proteins has the potential to support overall health and potentially aid in the management of uveitis. Nevertheless, individuals afflicted with uveitis must seek guidance from healthcare experts or registered dietitians to develop individualized nutrition plans that effectively target their unique requirements and medical circumstances.

Furthermore, in conjunction with nutritional interventions, the maintenance of a healthy lifestyle, which encompasses consistent physical activity and effective stress management, can be advantageous in the management of uveitis. Although uveitis is not curable on its own, nutrition can serve as a beneficial complement to medical interventions, potentially augmenting results and elevating the overall well-being of those afflicted with this difficult ocular condition. Further investigations in the domain of uveitis nutrition are expected to yield additional knowledge regarding the most effective dietary approaches to control and prevent the reoccurrence of this inflammatory ocular disorder.

THE END